CPR-AED
Cardiopulmonary Resuscitation (CPR)
and Automated External Defibrillation (A

AND **BASIC LIFE SUPPORT AND SAFE USE OF AN AED**

CW00400303

CONTENTS

Level 2 Award for CPR-AED | ISBN 978-1-908597-03-8
11th Edition : 2020-11-01

InstructUK Resources Ltd
Resources House, 10 Central Treviscoe, St Austell, Cornwall PL26 7QW

Tel: 0344 3320999
Web: www.instructuk.com

LEARNING OUTCOMES

Ofqual unit number: **J/503/1186**

SQA unit number: **U736 04**

Learning outcomes	Assessment criteria
1. Understand basic life support requirements	1.1 Describe the principles that underpin basic life support 1.2 Explain the circumstances under which resuscitation is Performed 1.3 Explain why early intervention is necessary 1.4 Describe different types of cardiopulmonary arrest
2. Be able to demonstrate basic life support techniques and automated external defibrillator use in line with current national guidelines	2.1 Demonstrate cardiopulmonary resuscitation 2.2 Demonstrate compression only resuscitation 2.3 Demonstrate the use of resuscitation barrier devices 2.4 Demonstrate how to manage a choking casualty 2.5 Demonstrate the use of an automated external defibrillator 2.6 Describe the differences when using an automated external defibrillator on a child
3. Be able to demonstrate post-resuscitation procedures	3.1 Demonstrate how to place a casualty in the recovery position 3.2 Identify the risks when placing a casualty in the recovery Position 3.3 Describe handover and reporting procedures
4. Be able to carry out basic user maintenance and troubleshoot problems with an automated external defibrillator breathing normally	4.1 Identify when a defibrillator battery requires changing 4.2 Identify when electrode pads need replacing 4.3 Demonstrate how to troubleshoot problems if the automated external defibrillator does not function correctly
5. Understand the safe use of an automated external defibrillator	5.1 Describe the safety considerations when using AED's

Coronary and heart disease (CHD) is the UK's biggest killer. Approximately 86,000 people die of a heart attack each year, which means that approximately every 6 minutes of every day, someone will die of a heart attack.

When someone goes into cardiac arrest, the heart will initially continue to beat, but in an uncoordinated, abnormal way. This severely abnormal, chaotic heart rhythm (arrhythmia) is known as ventricular fibrillation (VF).

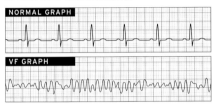

When suffering from VF, the heart is no longer able to pump blood to our most vital of organs, the brain, as well as other vital organs such as the lungs.

As a result of this, oxygen is not being transported from the lungs back to the heart, nor is it being transported around the body.

Death will occur in minutes if the heart's normal rhythm is not restored.

A very slight interruption to a normal heartbeat can lead to someone fainting, but ultimately it will lead to cardiac arrest and possible death if left untreated.

Causes, incidence, and risk factors

The most common cause of VF is a heart attack. However, VF can occur whenever the heart does not get enough oxygen, or if a person has other heart disorders.

Conditions that can lead to VF include:

- **Congenital heart disease**
- **Electrocution accidents or injury to the heart**
- **Heart attack**
- **Heart muscle disease or cardiomyopathy**
- **Heart surgery**
- **Ischemia (lack of oxygen to the heart muscle because of narrowed coronary arteries or shock)**
- **Sudden cardiac death, typically occurring in athletes after a trauma over the surface of the heart**

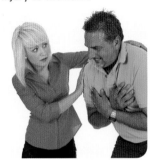

Most people with VF have no history of heart disease. However, many have risk factors for cardiovascular disease, such as:

- **Smoking**
- **Overweight**
- **Poor diet**
- **Lack of exercise**
- **High blood pressure**
- **Age**

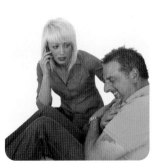

A casualty who has a VF episode will suddenly collapse or become unresponsive because the brain and muscles have stopped receiving blood from the heart.

The casualty's only chance of survival is with immediate treatment.

CPR could be enough for a small percentage of casualties. However, the chances of survival increase dramatically with a controlled electric shock from a defibrillator.

Automated External Defibrillators (AED's) will only shock the casualty if VF is present, or if its precursor is present, rapid ventricular tachycardia, or very rapid heart beat.

In the past, defibrillation was only ever offered by professional medical personnel. Over recent years this has changed with the development of AED's.

This means that with some basic training we can all use it, because it is automated.

AED's are becoming more common and can be found in many public places.

Although training is not mandatory, basic First Aid skills are an essential part of the whole process and, therefore, training is strongly recommended.

To emphasise the importance of defibrillation, the following graph will demonstrate that time really is of the essence.

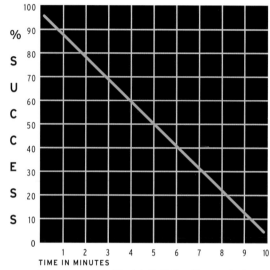

TIME IN MINUTES

For every minute without defibrillation, the casualty loses 10% chance of survival.

For each minute that defibrillation is delayed, the chances of your casualty recovering is reduced by 10%. Therefore, after about 10 minutes, your casualty will have little chance of surviving.

RESPONSIBILITIES

A First Aider has a number of responsibilities when dealing with an incident.

It is paramount that the incident is dealt with confidently and safely. The safety for all is important, including you, the casualty and any bystanders.

You must manage the incident and take control of the situation until professional medical help arrives and takes over. A bystander can be a great benefit to you, particularly if they are qualified in First Aid, so don't be afraid to summon help.

A bystander can make a telephone call, get a First Aid kit, return with the defibrillator if you have one, manage the crowd and traffic, and generally support you.

Your responsibilities can be broken up into the following categories:

- **Arrival at the scene**
- **Dealing with casualties**
- **Casualty communication**
- **Contacting the emergency services**
- **Prioritise the First Aid treatment**
- **Clearing up process and infection control**

ARRIVAL AT THE SCENE

Make the area safe and gather as much information about the incident as you can.

The history of the incident and any casualty information about their illness or injury could help you decide your course of initial treatment.

CONSENT

A responsive adult must agree to receive First Aid treatment. 'Expressed consent' means that the casualty gives their permission to receive care and treatment. To obtain consent, first identify yourself, tell them about your level of training and qualification and ask if it's ok to help them.

Implied consent means that permission to perform First Aid care on an unresponsive casualty is assumed. This is based on the idea that a reasonable person would give their permission to receive lifesaving treatment if they were able to.

When caring for vulnerable groups such as children and the elderly then consent must be gained from a parent, family member or legal guardian. When life-threatening situations exist and the parent, family member or legal guardian is not available, you must provide First Aid care based on implied consent.

Common sense

It is necessary to apply common sense. Never attempt skills that exceed your training. Always ask a responsive casualty for permission before giving care. Call for an ambulance immediately if no First Aid treatment is given. Once you have started First Aid, do not stop until medical help arrives and takes over from you.

Ensure you have help at hand.

You are almost certain to be feeling nervous and anxious yourself, but be as confident as you can, and take control of the situation.

DEALING WITH CASUALTIES

- Prioritise your treatment, particularly if you have multiple casualties
- Ensure safety for all
- Protect against contamination
- Be calm and confident
- Ensure that the appropriate emergency services have been called for

CASUALTY COMMUNICATION

Irrespective of the severity of the incident, your casualty could be in a state of shock and confusion. Therefore, your communication skills are critical in gaining their trust.

The groups that are most likely to be affected are children, the elderly, hearing impaired, visually impaired and non-English speaking casualties.

- Be honest about their condition, without exaggerating it
- Be careful of what you say which could distress them further
- Maintain eye contact when talking to them, and be aware of your body language. Their body language could tell you a lot about their condition
- Take your time when talking to them, particularly for the vulnerable groups such as the elderly and children
- Allow your casualty to explain how they are feeling. It could help you make a diagnosis enabling you to offer the right treatment
- In respect of their injury, avoid medical terms that they may not understand

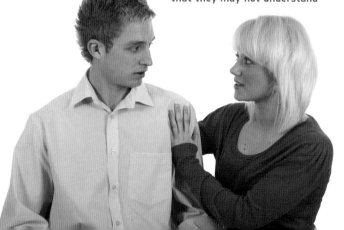

L I O N E L

CONTACTING THE EMERGENCY SERVICES

As soon as you have identified the extent of the injury, then it may be necessary to contact the emergency services. They can be contacted by dialling 999 or 112.

They will require vital information about the condition of the casualty so that the call can be prioritised.

Activate the speaker function on the phone to aid communication with the ambulance service.

They will also require specific details about the location of the incident. It is imperative that you have the full details of where you are, particularly if the premises are large and have multi-floors or other buildings to consider. Your bystander could manage this for you by meeting the emergency services and guiding them to the incident.

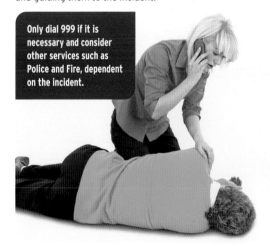

Only dial 999 if it is necessary and consider other services such as Police and Fire, dependent on the incident.

Remember **LIONEL** when making this call:

L Location

I Incident

O Other services

N Number of casualties

E Extent of injuries

L Location - repeat

PRIORITISE YOUR FIRST AID TREATMENT

- **Breathing** – deal with casualties who are not breathing normally first
- **Bleeding** – deal with any major bleeding and treat the casualty for shock
- **Burns/breaks** – treat burns and immobilise any bone injuries
- **Other conditions** – treat appropriately

There are many conditions that could be deemed as life-threatening which require medication, such as diabetes, asthma and anaphylaxis. Where possible, you can assist your casualty by offering them their own medication if they have it with them.

Remember your priorities. Ensure that their airway remains open and that they are breathing normally for themselves.

THE CLEARING UP PROCESS
AND INFECTION CONTROL

You must minimise the risk of infection from the outset when dealing with any incident. Similarly, when the casualty has been treated it is vital that all soiled dressings etc, are disposed of correctly.

- **Wash your hands and wear disposable gloves**
- **Avoid coughing and sneezing over the wound, and avoid touching it**
- **Dispose of all soiled dressings, including gloves, in an appropriately marked (orange/yellow) plastic bag**
- **Dispose of sharp items, including syringes and needles, in a purpose made sharps bin and dispose of it appropriately. It may mean taking it to your local hospital for correct disposal**

Rescuers should take appropriate safety precautions where feasible, especially if the casualty is known to have a serious infection such as tuberculosis (TB), severe acute respiratory distress syndrome (SARS) or coronavirus (COVID-19).

During any outbreak of a highly infectious condition, protective precautions for the rescuer are essential.

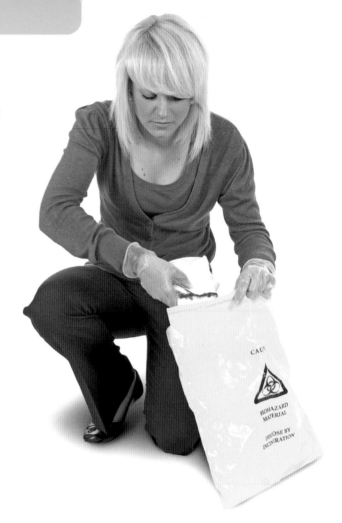

FIRST AID CONTAINERS

The minimum level of First Aid equipment is a suitably stocked and properly identified First Aid container.

Every employer should provide, for each work site, at least one First Aid container supplied with a sufficient quantity of First Aid materials suitable for the particular circumstances.

There is no mandatory list of items to be included in a First Aid container. The decision on what to provide, will be influenced by the findings of the First Aid needs assessment. As a guide, where work activities involve low hazards, a minimum stock of First Aid items might be:

- A leaflet giving general guidance on First Aid
- 20 individually wrapped sterile plasters (assorted sizes) appropriate to the type of work (hypoallergenic plasters can be provided if necessary)
- Two sterile eye pads
- Four individually wrapped triangular bandages, preferably sterile
- Six safety pins
- Two large sterile individually wrapped unmedicated wound dressings
- Six medium-sized individually wrapped un-medicated wound dressings
- A pair of disposable gloves

This is a suggested contents list only.

The contents of First Aid containers should be examined frequently and restocked soon after use. Sufficient supplies should be held in stock on site. Care should be taken to dispose of items safely once they reach their expiry date.

As from 30th June 2011 a new standard (BS-8599) came into effect that relates to First Aid kits, please visit the HSE website for further information, (see back page).

It is recommended that tablets and medicines should not be kept in the First Aid container.

ADDITIONAL FIRST-AID MATERIALS AND EQUIPMENT

The needs assessment may indicate that additional materials and equipment are required, for example scissors, burns dressings, adhesive tape, disposable aprons and individually wrapped moist wipes. They may be kept in the First Aid container if there is room, or stored separately.

If you have an AED, it would be a good idea to have a towel and a disposable razor at hand should you have to prepare the casualty's chest before applying the electrode pads to it.

If mains tap water is not readily available for eye irrigation, at least a litre of sterile water or sterile normal saline (0.9%) in sealed, disposable containers should be provided. Once the seal has been broken, containers should not be kept for re-use. Containers should not be used beyond their expiry date.

First Aid at work does not include giving tablets or medicines to treat illness. The only exception to this is where aspirin is used when giving First Aid to a casualty with a suspected heart attack in accordance with currently accepted First Aid practice. The view of the Health and Safety Executive (HSE), is that the administration of medication by a First Aider is not part of an Emergency First Aid at Work training course, but you can assist an individual in taking it, if it is their own medication. However, the one exception is heart attacks. Therefore, for heart attack management, the First Aider must be able to assist a casualty in taking 150-300 mg of chewable aspirin and to advise them to chew it, not swallow it, providing you are confident that the casualty is not allergic to it. If you are in any doubt, then you MUST NOT administer it. You must not administer an aspirin to anyone under the age of 16, and it should not be kept in the First Aid kit.

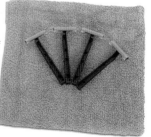

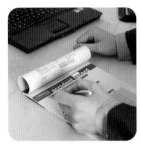

ACCIDENT AND INCIDENT REPORTING

Irrespective of the severity of the accident or incident, it is vital that all such occurrences be reported and filed by the employer.

Anyone can complete the accident book, and this book must comply with Data Protection legislation.

The accident book should be used as a useful reference for the purpose of ensuring that, where reasonably practicable, the same incident can be prevented from happening again.

An accident book can be purchased at most good book shops, or online from many First Aid supply shops.

The information that should be recorded includes:

- **The date, time and place of the incident**
- **Name and job of the injured or ill person**
- **Details of the injury/illness and what First Aid was given**
- **What happened to the casualty immediately afterwards?** (e.g. went back to work, went home, went to hospital)
- **Name and signature of the person reporting the incident**
- **The information must be kept in accordance with the Data Protection Act 2018**

Where the incident is of a severe nature, then the employer must comply with RIDDOR 2013.

RIDDOR is the law that requires employers, and other people in control of work premises, to report and keep records of:

- **Work-related accidents which cause death**
- **Work-related accidents which cause certain serious injuries (reportable injuries)**
- **Diagnosed cases of certain industrial diseases**
- **Certain 'dangerous occurrences' (incidents with the potential to cause harm)**

There are also special requirements for gas incidents.

Reporting certain incidents is a legal requirement. The report informs the enforcing authorities (HSE, local authorities and the Office for Rail Regulation (ORR)) about deaths, injuries, occupational diseases and dangerous occurrences, so they can identify where and how risks arise, and whether they need to be investigated.

Please visit **www.hse.gov.uk/riddor/** for full details of what is reportable.

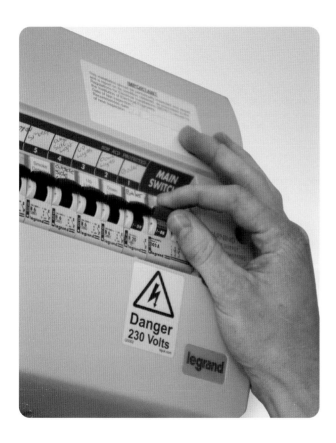

When confronted with any emergency situation, you need to take SHAPE!

 Safety and protection

You must ensure the safety for all. Ensure you are adequately protected against the risk of infection and any other adverse element such as chemicals and gases

 Hazards

Be aware of potential hazards such as traffic, chemicals, fire, gas, electricity etc

 Assess the situation

Before rushing in to deal with an incident, you must assess the situation that you are confronted with

 Prioritise

Ensure you prioritise the injuries, particularly if you have multiple casualties

 Environment

Pay attention to the environment around you, and do not take risks. Jumping into water to save a drowning victim is not a good idea if you can't swim!

Irrespective of the incident you are confronted with, you must carry out an initial assessment of the situation including your casualty.

This is popularly known as the primary survey.
The contents of this survey can be remembered easily by using the mnemonic **DR ABC**.

Dangers

The area must be safe before you offer your casualty any treatment. Safe for you primarily, not forgetting any bystanders and of course your casualty.

Failing to do this could result in you having more casualties to deal with, which could include yourself!

Response

Approach the casualty, ideally from their feet. This reduces the risk of the casualty hyper-extending their neck should they be responsive.

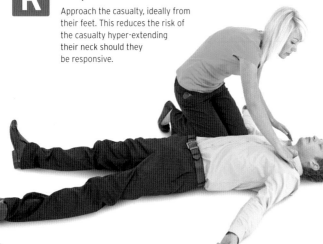

YOU CAN PERFORM A RESPONSIVE CHECK BY USING THE AVPU SCALE.

Alert   If they are fully responsive, then ascertain the extent of their injury and deal with it appropriately.

Voice - "Are you all right?"
If they are not alert, then see if they will respond to a voice command.

Place your hands on their shoulders and gently shake them.
If they don't respond to a voice command, then try shaking them gently by the shoulders. NB: do not shake them if you suspect a spinal or head injury.

Unresponsive
If there is no response at all, they must be deemed as being unresponsive.

If your casualty responds, leave them in the position in which you find them providing there is no further danger. Try to find out what is wrong with them and treat accordingly.

Call for professional medical help if it is needed and reassess them regularly.

If you are on your own, you should shout for help. Ideally you should never leave your casualty on their own.

A bystander can be a great benefit to you such as:

- **Calling for an ambulance**
- **Managing crowds and hazards**
- **Fetching the First Aid kit and defibrillator if you have one**
- **Consoling relatives and friends**
- **Helping you if they are trained to do so**
- **Cleaning up**
- **A support for you**

Airway

Turn the casualty onto their back and then open the airway using the head tilt and chin lift method:

- **Place your hand on their forehead and gently tilt their head back**
- **With two fingertips under the point of their chin, lift the chin to open the airway**
- **Be careful not to press on the fleshy part under the chin as it could restrict the airway**

Support their head in this position in order to perform a breathing check.

Breathing

Look, listen and feel for normal breathing for no more than 10 seconds.

Look   for chest movement
Listen at their mouth for breath sounds
Feel   for air on your cheek

In the first few minutes after cardiac arrest, a casualty may be barely breathing, or taking infrequent, noisy, gasps. This is often termed agonal breathing or gasping, and must not be confused with normal breathing.

If you have any doubt whether breathing is normal, act as if it is **not** normal and prepare to commence CPR.

The casualty who is **unresponsive** and **not breathing normally** is in cardiac arrest and requires CPR.

Immediately following cardiac arrest blood flow to the brain is reduced to virtually zero, which may cause seizure-like episodes that may be confused with epilepsy.

You should be suspicious of cardiac arrest with any casualty that presents seizure like symptoms and carefully assess whether they are breathing normally.

CPR for a non-breathing casualty

If your casualty **is not breathing normally**, then an ambulance must be summoned immediately. If you have a bystander at hand, then send them to make this important call so that you can commence Cardiopulmonary Resuscitation, or CPR without delay. (see page 18).

You can also ask your bystander to find and bring an Automated External Defibrillator (AED) to you, if one is available. However, if you are on your own, then you must call the emergency services yourself.

Stay with the casualty when making this call if possible. If you are able to, activate the speaker function on your phone to aid communication between you and the emergency services.

If your casualty is **breathing normally**, then treat any injuries accordingly and put them in the recovery position (see page 15).

Ask your bystander to summon an ambulance. If you are on your own, then make this call after placing them in the recovery position.

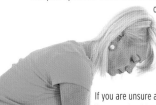

Ensure that you monitor their breathing whilst in the recovery position.

If you are unsure about the extent of the injury, then you should perform a top-to-toe survey before placing them in the recovery position (see page 15).

 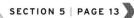

As soon as you have completed your primary survey, and you have established that your casualty is breathing normally, you must then move on to the secondary assessment in order to determine the extent of their injury or illness, irrespective of whether they are responsive or not.

In order to make a diagnosis of their condition, there are three key factors to consider. By making this diagnosis correctly, it should determine the treatment you offer them. In all cases, your priority is to maintain an open airway and to ensure that they are breathing normally.

History

- Ask your casualty or bystanders what happened
- Examine the environment for obvious signs relating to the incident
- Ask your casualty about their condition. Do they have their own medication? Has it happened before? Where does it hurt? How painful is it?
- Ask the casualty their name. Is there any family present that could answer the questions about their condition?

Signs

- What can you see in respect of the injury or condition?
- Use all your other senses. What can you smell, hear and feel?

Symptoms

This is how the casualty will be feeling, ask them how they are feeling.

- Communication is very important to ascertain the extent of their injury/illness
- Continue to question their well-being throughout your assessment as they may have deteriorated which may influence your decision on the appropriate treatment

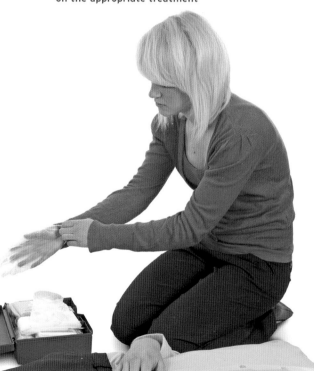

The recovery position

If your casualty is unresponsive, but breathing normally, then your priority is to ensure that their airway is not compromised in any way and that it remains open.

Rather than leaving them on their back, or in a slumped position, then an effective way of achieving this is to place them in the recovery position.

Whilst the casualty remains in this position, it will allow vomit to drain from the mouth and prevent them from rolling onto their back should you have to leave them.

1 Remove the casualty's glasses, if present

2 Kneel beside the casualty and make sure that both their legs are straight

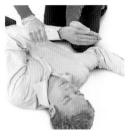
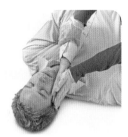

3 Place the arm nearest to you out at a right angle to their body, elbow bent with the hand palm-up. Do not force the arm, let it fall naturally, but close to this position

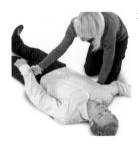

Suspected spinal injury
If you suspect a spinal injury and you cannot maintain an open airway in the position you found them, care must be taken in moving them.
Keep the casualty's back straight and support the head throughout. It would be extremely useful to have help in moving the casualty. The trained person should assume control when moving them.

4 Bring the far arm across the chest, and hold the back of the hand against their cheek nearest to you

5 With your other hand, grasp the far leg just above the knee and pull it up, keeping the foot on the ground

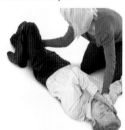

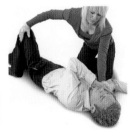
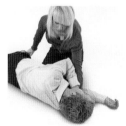

6 Keeping their hand pressed against their cheek, pull on the far leg to roll them towards you onto their side with their head supported all the way

 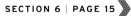

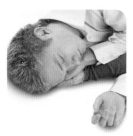

7 Tilt the head back to make sure that the airway remains open

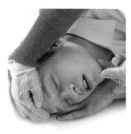

8 If necessary, adjust the hand under their cheek to keep the head tilted and facing downwards to allow liquid material to drain from the mouth

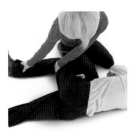

9 Adjust the upper leg so that both the hip and knee are bent at right angles

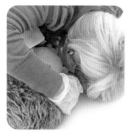

10 Check breathing regularly

11 **If you have a bystander available to you, then this is the time to send them to call for an ambulance ensuring they have all the appropriate information, and in particular, the condition of the casualty**

12 **If you have no bystander, you must call for an ambulance yourself**

If they have to be kept in the recovery position for **more than 30 minutes** turn them to the opposite side to relieve the pressure on the lower arm.

You must continue to monitor their breathing whilst waiting for the emergency services to take over. If they stop breathing normally, then you must call the emergency services with an update and commence CPR immediately.

It will also be worth monitoring and noting other changes such as colouration of the skin, their temperature and responsiveness levels.

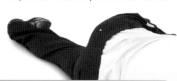

Pregnant women

Always put an unresponsive pregnant woman in recovery position on her **left side**.

This prevents compression of the Inferior vena cava (large vein) by the uterus, which could be **fatal** for both the mother and the child.

Our ability to breathe is thanks to our respiratory system which is made up primarily of our airways and our lungs.

We are able to breathe in and out spontaneously providing we have air to breathe and the airways are open.

COMPOSITION OF AIR

Air breathed in

- Nitrogen - 78%
- Oxygen - 21%
- Argon and other gases - 1%

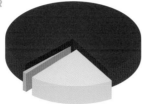

When we breathe in the diaphragm contracts and flattens, the ribs are elevated, and as negative pressure is produced in the chest cavity, there is increased pressure in the abdomen. This draws air into the lungs to equalise the pressure.

We exhale when the diaphragm relaxes and the chest wall and lung tissue returns to their original size.

Respiration is achieved through the mouth, nose, trachea, lungs, and diaphragm. Oxygen enters the respiratory system through the mouth and the nose. The oxygen then passes through the larynx (where speech sounds are produced) and the trachea which is a tube that enters the chest cavity. In the chest cavity, the trachea splits into two smaller tubes called the bronchi. Each bronchus then divides again forming the bronchioles. These bronchial tubes lead directly into the lungs where they divide into many smaller tubes which connect to tiny sacs called alveoli. The average adult's lungs contain about 600 million of these spongy, air-filled sacs that are surrounded by capillaries. The inhaled oxygen passes

into the alveoli and then enters the capillaries (diffusion) into the arterial blood which is taken back to the heart for circulating around the body.

Meanwhile, the waste-rich blood from the veins releases its carbon dioxide into the alveoli. The carbon dioxide follows the same path out of the lungs when you breathe out.

Approximately 25% of the available oxygen in each breath is used, as our body can only cope with so much each time we breathe in.

Carbon dioxide and other non-essential gases are breathed out and the whole process is repeated between 10 - 20 times per minute for an average adult.

The Respiratory System

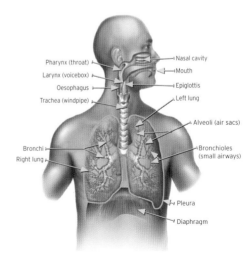

Pharynx (throat)
Larynx (voicebox)
Oesophagus
Trachea (windpipe)
Nasal cavity
Mouth
Epiglottis
Left lung
Alveoli (air sacs)
Bronchi
Right lung
Bronchioles (small airways)
Pleura
Diaphragm

Cardiopulmonary resuscitation (CPR) is an emergency procedure which is attempted in an effort to return life to a person who is not breathing normally for themselves.

This procedure combines chest compressions with rescue breaths. The chest compression replaces the heart's ability to pump oxygenated blood around the body, particularly to the vital organs such as the brain.

Rescue breathing provides the casualty, who is unable to breathe normally for themselves, valuable oxygen that is transported around the body by the chest compressions.

Without oxygen, brain damage can occur within three minutes. Therefore, your immediate action is paramount.

Referring back to Primary Survey,
i.e. DR ABC, then you will have established that your casualty is not breathing normally.

Your immediate action now is to contact the emergency services and ask for an ambulance, ensuring that you state that your casualty is not breathing normally.

If you have a bystander at hand, then send them to make this important call. You can also ask your bystander to find and bring an Automated External Defibrillator (AED) to you, if one is available.

However, if you are on your own, then you **must** call the emergency services yourself. Stay with the casualty when making this call if possible.

If you are able to, activate the speaker function on your phone to aid communication between you and the emergency services.

Commence CPR without delay.

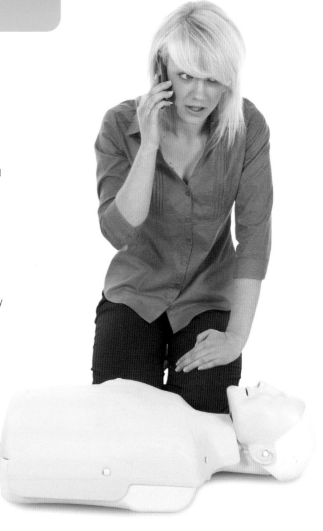

1. START WITH 30 CHEST COMPRESSIONS

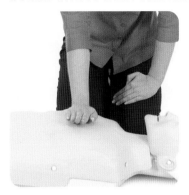

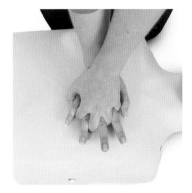

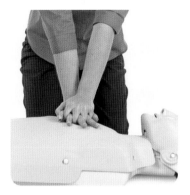

- **Kneel by the side of your casualty**
- **Place the heel of one hand in the centre of the casualty's chest** (which is the lower half of the casualty's breastbone (sternum)

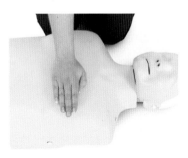

- **Place the heel of your other hand on top of the first hand**
- **Interlock the fingers of your hands and ensure that pressure is not applied over their ribs. Do not apply any pressure over the upper abdomen or the bottom end of the sternum**
- **Position yourself vertically above their chest and, with your arms straight, press down on the sternum approximately 5cm (But not more than 6cm)**

- **After each compression, release all the pressure on the chest without losing contact between your hands and the sternum. Do not lean on the chest.**
- **Repeat 30 chest compressions at a speed of 100 - 120 compressions per minute with as few interruptions as possible**
- **Compression and release should take an equal amount of time**

In most circumstances it will be possible to identify the correct hand position for chest compressions, without removing the casualty's clothes. If you are in any doubt, then remove outer clothing.

2. GIVE 2 RESCUE BREATHS After 30 chest compressions open the airway again using head tilt and chin lift.

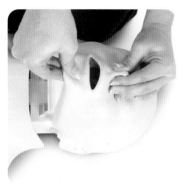 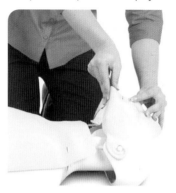 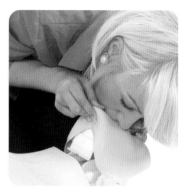

- Pinch the soft part of their nose closed, using the index finger and thumb of your hand on their forehead
- Allow their mouth to open, but maintain chin lift
- Take a normal breath and place your lips around their mouth, making sure that you have a good seal
- Blow steadily into their mouth whilst watching for their chest to rise, taking about one second as in normal breathing; this is an effective rescue breath

- Maintaining head tilt and chin lift, watch for their chest to fall as air comes out
- Take another normal breath and blow into the casualty's mouth once more to achieve a total of two effective rescue breaths. Do not interrupt compressions by more than 10 seconds to deliver two breaths. Then return your hands without delay to the correct position on the sternum and give a further 30 chest compressions

If the initial rescue breath of each sequence does not make the chest rise as in normal breathing, then, before your next attempt:

- Check the casualty's mouth and remove any visible obstruction
- Re-check that there is adequate head tilt and chin lift
- Do not attempt more than two breaths each time before returning to chest compressions

In order to reduce the risk of cross-contamination, there are various protective shields and masks available that will significantly reduce this risk. For more information about infection control please see page 12.

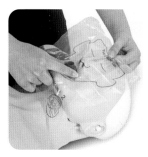 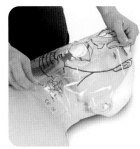 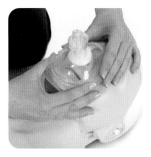 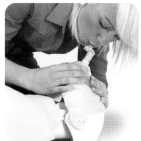

Repeat 30 compressions and 2 breaths until

- **A health professional tells you to stop**
- **The casualty is definitely waking up, moving, opening their eyes and breathing normally**
- **You become exhausted**

It is rare for CPR alone to restart the heart. Unless you are certain the casualty has recovered, continue with CPR.

Signs the casualty has recovered include:

- **Waking up**
- **Moving**
- **Opens eyes**

AND

- **They start breathing normally again**

Be prepared to restart CPR immediately if the casualty deteriorates.

It must be emphasised that if you are unable to give rescue breaths for whatever reason, then you must continue with chest-compression-only CPR.

If there is more than one rescuer present, another should take over CPR about every 1-2 minutes to prevent fatigue.

Ensure the minimum of delay during the changeover of rescuers and do not interrupt chest compressions.

IF YOU HAVE ACCESS TO AN AED

As soon as it arrives, switch it on and attach the electrode pads on the casualty's chest. Follow the voice prompts. If more than one rescuer is present, CPR should be continued whilst the electrode pads are being attached to the chest.

THE CHAIN OF SURVIVAL

It is critical that you follow this chain when you are dealing with a casualty who is not breathing normally.

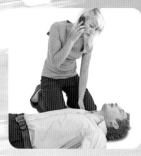 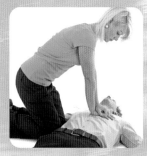 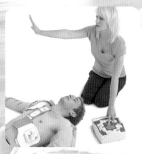 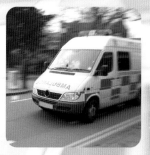

Early recognition and call for help

Recognise those at risk of cardiac arrest, and call for help in the hope that early treatment can prevent arrest.

Early CPR

Start CPR to buy time until medical help arrives.

Early defibrillation

Defibrillators give an electric shock to re-organise the rhythm of the heart.

Defibrillation within 3–5 minutes of cardiac arrest can produce survival rates as high as 50-70%.

Each minute of delay to defibrillation reduces the probability of survival to hospital discharge by 10%.

Post-resuscitation care

Provide professional help in order to restore the quality of life.

ADULT BASIC LIFE SUPPORT

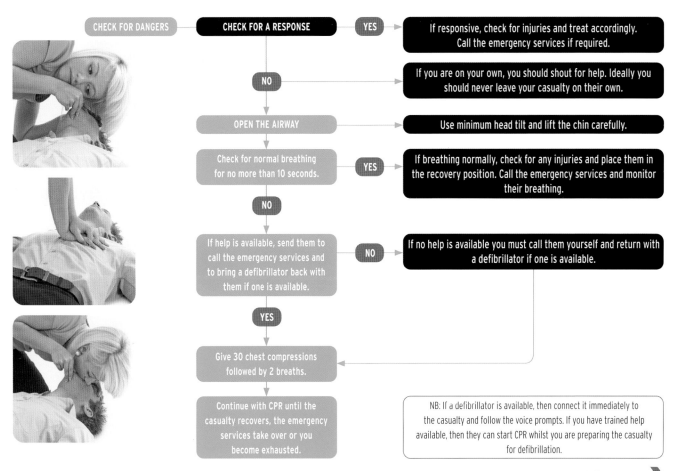

CHECK FOR DANGERS → **CHECK FOR A RESPONSE** → **YES**

If responsive, check for injuries and treat accordingly. Call the emergency services if required.

NO

If you are on your own, you should shout for help. Ideally you should never leave your casualty on their own.

OPEN THE AIRWAY

Use minimum head tilt and lift the chin carefully.

Check for normal breathing for no more than 10 seconds. → **YES**

If breathing normally, check for any injuries and place them in the recovery position. Call the emergency services and monitor their breathing.

NO

If help is available, send them to call the emergency services and to bring a defibrillator back with them if one is available. → **NO**

If no help is available you must call them yourself and return with a defibrillator if one is available.

YES

Give 30 chest compressions followed by 2 breaths.

Continue with CPR until the casualty recovers, the emergency services take over or you become exhausted.

NB: If a defibrillator is available, then connect it immediately to the casualty and follow the voice prompts. If you have trained help available, then they can start CPR whilst you are preparing the casualty for defibrillation.

CHOKING

There are many factors that can contribute to a respiratory disorder, including asthma, hypoxia, smoke inhalation and choking.

Choking is probably the most common of the disorders and probably the most distressing to suffer and to deal with.

Your immediate treatment is required. Should your casualty become unresponsive as a result of choking, then you will have to start resuscitation.

Recognition of someone choking

- Difficulty in speaking and breathing
- Coughing or gagging
- Clutching at the throat and pointing to the mouth
- Pale, grey/blue skin tone in the later stages (cyanosis)
- Ultimately - unresponsiveness

If your casualty shows signs of a mild or partial airway obstruction then:

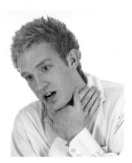

- Encourage them to continue coughing, but do nothing else at this stage
- Stay calm and offer plenty of encouragement and reassurance

Treatment for a severe airway obstruction for an adult

- Encourage them to cough
- Check their mouth and remove any obvious obstruction

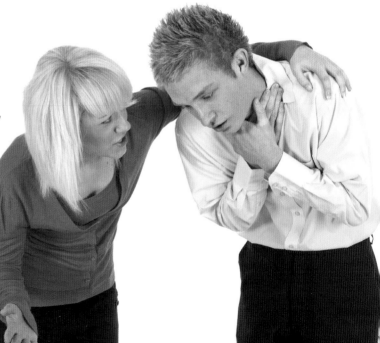

Bend them forward and give up to five back blows

- Stand to the side and slightly behind your casualty

- Support the chest with one hand and lean them forward so that when the obstructing object is dislodged it comes out of the mouth rather than to go further down the airway

- Give up to five sharp blows between their shoulder blades with the heel of your other hand

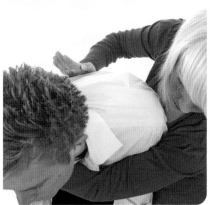

Check to see if each back blow has relieved the airway obstruction. The aim is to relieve the obstruction with each blow rather than to give all five unnecessarily.

Continued on page 26.

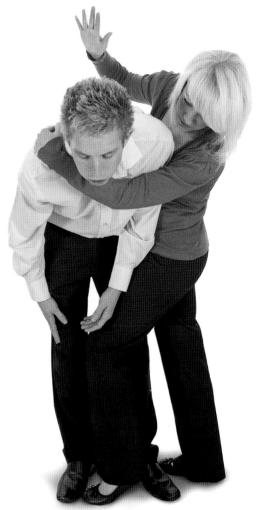

Give them up to five abdominal thrusts

- Stand behind your casualty and put both arms round the upper part of their abdomen

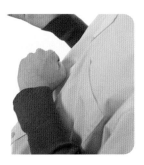 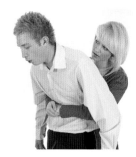 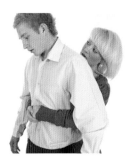 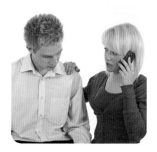

- Lean them forward
- Clench your fist and place it between the umbilicus (navel) and the bottom end of their sternum (breastbone)

- Grasp this hand with your other hand and pull sharply inwards and upwards
- Repeat up to five times

- Check to see if each abdominal thrust has relieved the airway obstruction. The aim is to relieve the obstruction with each thrust rather than to give all five unnecessarily

If you have performed abdominal thrusts on a casualty, they must be sent to hospital to be examined for any internal injuries.

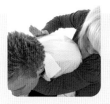

If the obstruction cannot be removed after the **first cycle** of back blows and abdominal thrusts, then you must call for an ambulance immediately.

Repeat the process of up to five back blows followed by up to five abdominal thrusts until the casualty recovers, or the emergency medical services take over from you.

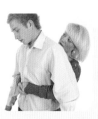

If your casualty becomes unresponsive, then help them to the floor onto their back, call 999/112 and commence CPR immediately.

Before each rescue breath attempt, check in the mouth for any visible obstruction that can be removed easily without having to sweep the mouth with your fingers.

WHAT IS AN AED?

An automated external defibrillator (AED) is a lightweight, portable device that delivers a controlled electric shock through the chest to the heart, via two electrodes that are fixed to the casualty's chest. The AED is able to detect the rhythm of the heart, similar to that of an electrocardiogram (ECG), and it can deliver a shock that can reverse ventricular fibrillation (VF) and therefore restore a normal heart rhythm.

The quicker an AED is attached to the casualty, the greater the chances are of survival.

Self testing

Periodically, AED's will self-test themselves to ensure that that they are fit for purpose.

Most will have a green and red light indicator. Some will have an audible alarm.

The red light will indicate there is a problem, and a green light indicates that it is ready for use. The test is generally based on the condition of the battery, that it is sufficiently charged. Some will also check the condition of the electro pads.

On/off button

Some AED's will switch themselves on as soon as the lid is removed or opened. Some will have an 'on/off' button.

Voice prompts

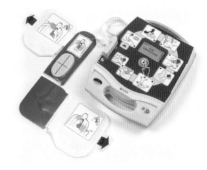

All AED's will have a voice prompt which you must follow. As soon as it is switched on, the AED will start to talk to you! Commands such as "connect electrodes", "analysing – do not touch the patient" and "shock advised – do not touch the patient" are typical commands.

Display window

Some AED's will have an LCD display, showing voice prompt messages. This can be particularly useful for operatives who are hard of hearing.

Metronome

Some will have a built-in metronome when administering chest compressions to ensure that the casualty's chest is being compressed at the right speed. Some will even tell you to 'push harder' and offer you a congratulatory message!

The electrodes or pads

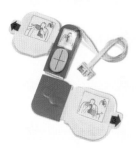

These can be provided as two separate pads, or as a one-piece pad. The correct positioning is vital, and there will generally be a display on the pads where they should be positioned. In order to adhere to the casualty's chest, the pad/s will be adhesive and a film protecting this adhesive will have to be removed. There is a shelf life and the pads should be checked to ensure they are still in date. If the packaging is damaged in any way, they should be replaced. Ideally, you should have a spare set available to you.

ANALYSING VARIATIONS

All AED's will have an analysing facility built-in. Some will self-analyse with no intervention necessary from the operative, whilst others will invite you to push the analyse button.

Irrespective of the type, you must ensure that no-one is touching the casualty.

THE CHARGE VARIATIONS

An AED can shock a casualty from as little as 50 joules for children and up to 360 joules for an adult. Some will shock the casualty with a monophasic charge ie: an electrical charge is passed from one electrode to another in one direction. A biphasic charge will pass from one electrode to another and then is reversed. The number of joules is reduced as a result of biphasic, causing less potential damage to the heart.

EMBEDDED PROTOCOLS

All AED's will have an embedded protocol or procedure for defibrillation. This protocol can change from time to time by authoritative bodies such as the Resuscitation Council UK and the European Resuscitation Council. When there is a change, the AED's should be upgraded to reflect this change. Most AED's can be re-programmed to accommodate this.

The AED is generally changed by the manufacturer or by yourself, with software provided by them.

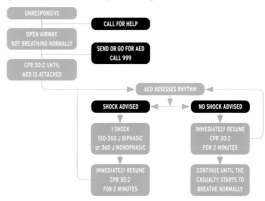

RECORDING THE PROCESS OF DEFIBRILLATION

Many AED's will be able to record the process from start to finish. Information about time, number of shocks given, rhythm of the heart, number of compressions given etc is recorded which can then be subsequently printed off.

This is invaluable information for the medical professionals in post-resuscitation care.

AED BATTERIES

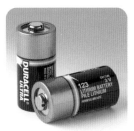

You must ensure that the batteries in your AED are fully charged and ready to go at a moment's notice.

The batteries will vary from one AED to another. Some have a rechargeable lithium battery that can only be supplied by the manufacturer or AED suppliers. Some will have a non-rechargeable lithium battery. Some will be fitted with consumer lithium batteries that can be purchased at most large local stores.

What is important is that the batteries are fully charged at all times. It may be wise to keep a spare battery, or set of batteries.

PAEDIATRIC FACILITY

Most manufacturers will have specially designed pads for defibrillating children. They will generally offer an automatically reduced electrical charge.

Generally speaking a child is deemed as being from the age of 1 to 8, or up to 25kg in weight (55lbs). Any young person aged from 8 upwards, should be treated as an adult for the purposes of defibrillation.

An infant is aged from birth to 1 year old. Some AED manufacturers will be able to provide pads for this age group. The use of an AED is not recommended for this age group. However, if an AED is the only defibrillator available, then it should be considered particularly if you have the specially modified pads.

FAMILIARISATION WITH YOUR OWN AED

You will have probably realised that there are many variations in AED's. It is important to familiarise yourself with your own AED in respect of the controls, batteries and electrodes/pads.

As far as training is concerned, your instructor may well be using a different AED training unit from the one that you are familiar with. As long as the protocols that are embedded in the unit are up-to-date, then this is fine.

If you are in any doubt about the specification of your AED, consult your manufacturer.

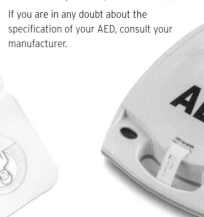

DEFIBRILLATION WITH AN AED

If your casualty is in a wet environment, then move them to a dry area and ensure that they are not in contact with anything metal.

When the AED arrives, you must immediately unpack it and prepare to fix the pads to the casualty. If you have trained help, then allow them to continue with CPR until you are ready. If not, then stop CPR and unpack it yourself.

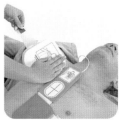

If your casualty is wearing a wired bra, then this must be removed or cut through to expose the chest, particularly the area where the pads are to be fixed. Similarly, if your casualty is wearing jewellery that may come into contact with the pads, then it must be removed.

The majority of pads will be clearly marked on where they should be fixed. Depending on the make and model of the AED, the pads will generally come as two separate pads. Some will come as a single pad. Ensure that the film that is protecting the sticky pads is removed.

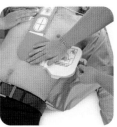

If your casualty has a pacemaker fitted, then ensure that the pads are placed at least 10cms away from it.

Do not place the pads directly on top of it. A pacemaker should be clearly identifiable, from a scar or what appears to be a small plate under the skin.

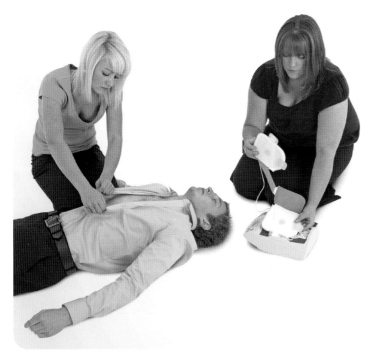

> It may be necessary to prepare the casualty's chest in order for the pads to adhere. Do not waste valuable time shaving inappropriately.

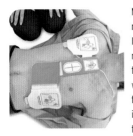

Most AED pads are labelled left and right, or carry a picture of the placement. It does not matter if these pads are reversed. What is important is that should they be placed the wrong way round, they must be left in place because the adhesive may well be removed or compromised if you swap them around.

In respect of switching the AED on, they will vary from one AED to another. Some will switch themselves on as soon as the lid is removed or opened. Others will have a button to press to switch it on.

It is important that you familiarise yourself with the AED you have.

All AED's will have a voice prompt and it is important that you follow these prompts.

Some AED's will also have a screen giving you the commands. This can be a very useful aid for those who are hard of hearing.

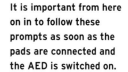

It is important from here on in to follow these prompts as soon as the pads are connected and the AED is switched on.

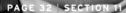

The AED will need to analyse the heart's rhythm. You will be prompted to ensure that no-one is touching the casualty, including yourself. Anyone touching the casualty could have an adverse effect on detecting the correct rhythm of your casualty's heart.

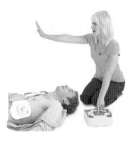

Dependent on the model you have, analysis will automatically happen, or you may have to push the 'Analyse' button.

You have to take control of the situation and move people away from the casualty.

Your next prompt could be to shock the casualty. Your AED may do this automatically, or you may have to press the 'Shock' button.

Again, manage the situation and ensure that no-one is touching the casualty.

Keep following the prompts from the AED.

If you are prompted to commence CPR, then quality CPR is important.

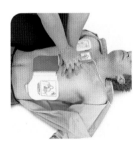

Ensure that you compress at the right depth (5-6cms) and at the right speed (100-120 chest compressions per minute).

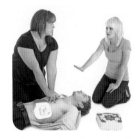

In essence you must continue with CPR until the AED tells you to stop to either analyse the casualty's heart rhythm, or it decides that a shock should be given.

Under the current resuscitation guidelines, you will be administering CPR for two minutes before the AED will prompt you to stop in order for it to analyse the heart's rhythm.

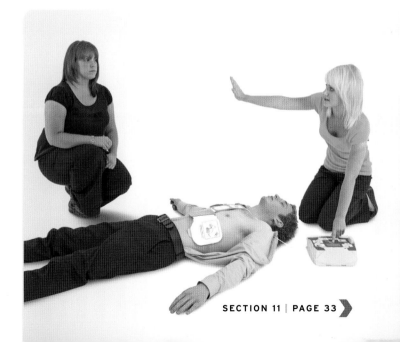

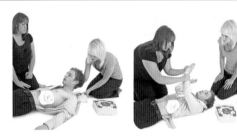 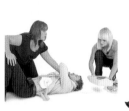 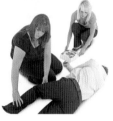 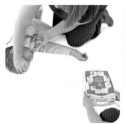 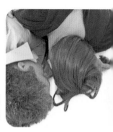

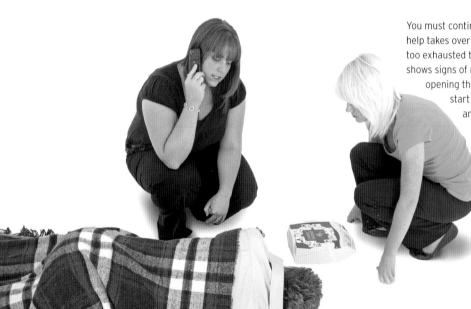

You must continue to follow the prompts until professional medical help takes over from you, your casualty recovers, or you become too exhausted to continue. Recovery will mean that your casualty shows signs of regaining responsiveness, such as coughing, opening their eyes, speaking or moving purposefully AND they start to breathe normally for themselves. To ensure they are breathing normally, conduct a breathing check.

If you are confident that they are breathing normally, place them in the recovery position with the pads attached and connected to the AED.

You must continue to monitor their breathing until professional medical help arrives and takes over from you.

PAEDIATRIC DEFIBRILLATION

The protocol for paediatric defibrillation is the same as that for an adult.

Most manufacturers are able to offer you specially modified pads for children, that means you can use the same AED for adults and children. However, what it is important to know are the differences between adults, children and infants in respect of your Basic Life Support procedures. This section deals with those differences.

The term paediatric refers to children and infants (babies). A child is deemed as being aged from 1 to the onset of puberty and an infant being aged under 1 year old.

Many manufacturers refer to children as being from the age of 1 to 8. If you are in doubt about whether a child has reached puberty, then use the age of 8 as your guide. Any child that is older than 8 years of age should be treated as an adult, and the adult protocols for CPR and defibrillation should be adopted.

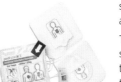

Most manufacturers will have specially adapted pads to accommodate a child.

The pads for children are generally smaller. When they are connected to the AED, the device will recognise them and administer the appropriate electric shock, which is generally a reduced charge.

Defibrillation is not recommended for infants unless the manufacturer of the AED you have has specially adapted pads that can be connected. You must check with your supplier to see if pads are available.

If you have an incident to deal with that involves a child or infant, then you should carry out a primary survey as defined in section 5.

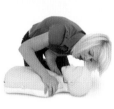 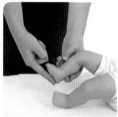 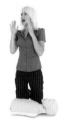 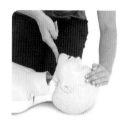 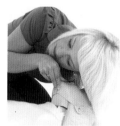 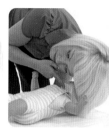

PAEDIATRIC CPR

The principles of resuscitation, is the same as with an adult, but with a few subtle differences.

1 Check for dangers

2 Check for a response. Gently stimulate the child and ask loudly "are you alright?"

Do not shake infants or children with a suspected spinal injury. You can stimulate an infant by rubbing the soles of their feet with your finger to see if there is a response.

If the child responds by answering, crying or moving:

- Leave the child in the position in which you find them (providing they are not in further danger)
- Check their condition and call for help
- Reassess them regularly

3 If you are on your own, you should shout for help.

The casualty who is **unresponsive** and **not breathing normally** is in cardiac arrest and requires CPR.

Immediately following cardiac arrest blood flow to the brain is reduced to virtually zero, which may cause seizure-like episodes that may be confused with epilepsy.

You should be suspicious of cardiac arrest with any casualty that presents seizure like symptoms and carefully assess whether they are breathing normally.

CHILD AND INFANT

4 Open the airway

Turn the child/infant onto their back and open the airway using head tilt and chin lift:

- Place your hand on their forehead and gently tilt their head back
- With your fingertip(s) under the point of their chin, lift the chin. Use one finger for an infant and take care not to over-extend the neck when tilting the head back
- Do not push on the soft tissues under the chin as this may block the airway

5 Check for normal breathing

Keeping the airway open, look, listen and feel for normal breathing by putting your face close to their face and looking along their chest:

- Look for chest movements
- Listen at their nose and mouth for breath sounds
- Feel for air movement on your cheek. In the first few minutes after a cardiac arrest a child/infant may be taking slow infrequent gasps. Look, listen and feel for no more than 10 seconds before deciding. If you have any doubt whether breathing is normal, act as if it is not normal

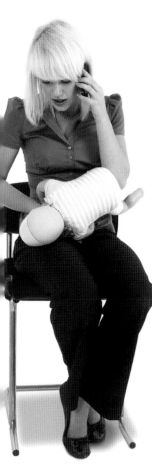

6a   If they are breathing normally:

- **Turn them on their side into the recovery position**
  NB: Consider the history of trauma and spinal injury before putting them in the recovery position.
  (see pages 43 and 44 for child and infant recovery position)

- **Send your bystander to go for help and call 999/112 for an ambulance.**

  If you are on your own, then make this call yourself. If you are able to do so, take the casualty with you

- **Continue to monitor their breathing**

6b If they are not breathing normally, or if it is absent:

- **Carefully remove any obvious airway obstruction**

You are on your own

- **Give five initial rescue breaths, followed by 1 minute of CPR ie: approximately 2 cycles of 30 chest compressions followed by 2 rescue breaths, and then call 999/112 for an ambulance and return with the defibrillator if you have one.**

  Upon your return, unpack and connect the AED to your casualty and follow the voice prompts. If you don't have an AED, then continue with 30 chest compressions followed by 2 breaths and repeat 30:2 until professional medical help takes over, your casualty recovers*, or you become too exhausted to continue.

You have help available

- **Send them to call for an ambulance immediately and to return with the AED if you have one**

  You must give 5 initial breaths, followed by continuous CPR ie: 30 chest compressions followed by 2 rescue breaths and then repeat 30:2 until the AED arrives. Unpack and connect the AED to your casualty and follow the voice prompts. If you don't have an AED, then you must continue with CPR ie: 30:2 after giving the 5 initial breaths, until professional medical help takes over, your casualty recovers*, or you become too exhausted to continue.

- * Recovery means that the casualty starts to show signs of regaining responsiveness, such as:

  - Waking up

  - Moving

  - Opens eyes

  AND

  - **They start breathing normally again**

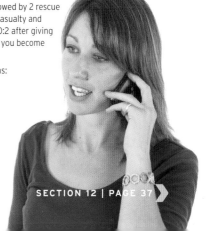

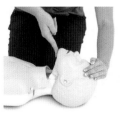
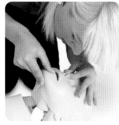
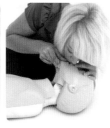
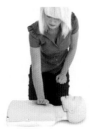
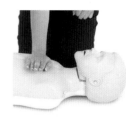
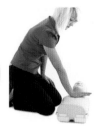

CHILD CPR

Technique for giving rescue breaths for a child over 1 year:

- Ensure head tilt and chin lift
- Pinch the soft part of their nose closed with the index finger and thumb of your hand on their forehead
- Open their mouth a little, but maintain the chin lift
- Take a breath and place your lips around their mouth, making sure that you have a good seal
- Blow steadily into their mouth over 1 second, sufficient to make the chest rise visibly. This is the same time period as in adult practice
- Maintaining head tilt and chin lift, take your mouth away and watch for their chest to fall as air comes out
- Take another breath and repeat this sequence four more times. Identify the effectiveness by seeing that their chest has risen and fallen in a similar fashion to the movement produced by a normal breath

Technique for giving chest compressions for children aged over 1 year:

- Place the heel of one hand on the lower half of the breastbone (sternum)
- Lift the fingers to ensure that pressure is not applied over their ribs
- Position yourself vertically above their chest and, with your arm straight, compress the sternum to depress it by at least one-third of the depth of the chest which is approximately 5cms
- Release the pressure completely, then repeat at a rate of 100-120 compressions per minute

For larger children, or for small rescuers, this may be achieved most easily by using both hands with the fingers interlocked

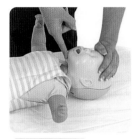

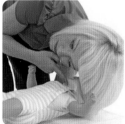

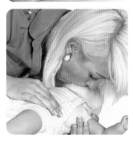

INFANT CPR

Technique for giving rescue breaths for an infant:

- Ensure a neutral position of the head (as an infant's head is usually flexed when on their back and face up (supine), this may require some extension) and apply chin lift

- Take a breath and cover the mouth and nose of the infant with your mouth, making sure you have a good seal. If both the nose and mouth cannot be covered in the older infant, then attempt to seal only the infant's nose or mouth with your mouth (if the nose is used, close the lips to prevent air escape and vice versa)

- Blow steadily into their mouth over 1 second, sufficient to make the chest rise visibly. This is the same time period as in adult practice

- Maintain head position and chin lift, take your mouth away, and watch for their chest to fall as air comes out

- Take another breath and repeat this sequence four more times

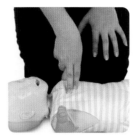

Technique for giving chest compressions for infants:

- Place the tips of 2 fingers in the centre of the breastbone (sternum)

- Compress the sternum to depress it by at least one-third of the depth of the chest which is approximately 4cms

- Release the pressure completely, then repeat at a rate of 100-120 compressions per minute

For both infants and children, if you have difficulty achieving an effective breath, the airway may be obstructed:

- Open their mouth and remove any visible obstruction. Do not perform a blind finger sweep

- Ensure that there is adequate head tilt and chin lift but also that the neck is not over extended

- Make up to 5 attempts to achieve effective breaths. If this is still unsuccessful, move on to chest compressions

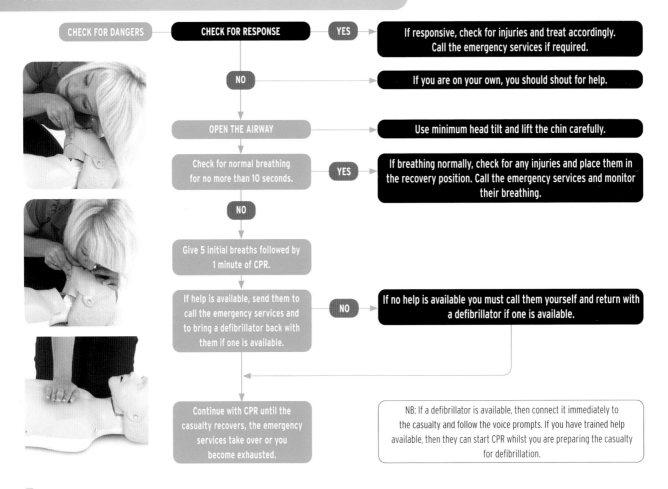

CHECK FOR DANGERS

CHECK FOR RESPONSE → **YES** → If responsive, check for injuries and treat accordingly. Call the emergency services if required.

NO → If you are on your own, you should shout for help.

OPEN THE AIRWAY → Use minimum head tilt and lift the chin carefully.

Check for normal breathing for no more than 10 seconds. → **YES** → If breathing normally, check for any injuries and place them in the recovery position. Call the emergency services and monitor their breathing.

NO

Give 5 initial breaths followed by 1 minute of CPR.

If help is available, send them to call the emergency services and to bring a defibrillator back with them if one is available. → **NO** → If no help is available you must call them yourself and return with a defibrillator if one is available.

Continue with CPR until the casualty recovers, the emergency services take over or you become exhausted.

NB: If a defibrillator is available, then connect it immediately to the casualty and follow the voice prompts. If you have trained help available, then they can start CPR whilst you are preparing the casualty for defibrillation.

SAFETY

- If supplementary oxygen is being used for the purposes of resuscitation, then remove the mask from the casualty and move it along with the oxygen tank, at least one metre away from the casualty. This also applies to any other flammable gases, chemicals and explosives

- Ensure that the casualty is removed from direct contact with water or metal, and check that there is no direct path of water between you and the casualty

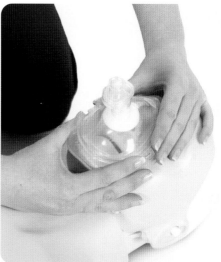

- Ensure that no-one is touching the casualty when the AED is analysing or administering a shock to them

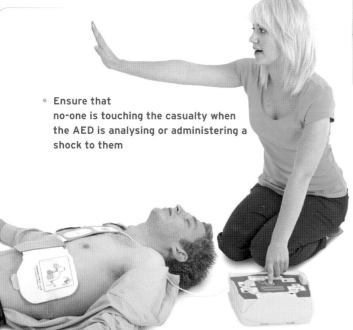

- Reduce the risk of cross-contamination by using a face-shield or mask when giving your casualty rescue breaths during CPR

> Never use a 'live' unit for training, unless it can be modified to do so

STORAGE

- AED's should be stored in an immediately accessible area
- Don't store them in a locked area, as this could cause a delay
- Ensure that all rescuers are aware of the location
- Cabinets and wall brackets are available from most manufacturers
- The storage area should be dry and relatively dust free

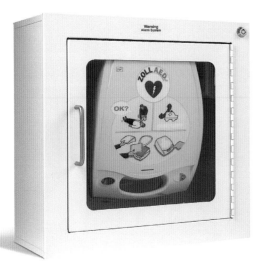

CONSIDERATIONS

- Follow the voice prompts at all times
- Quality CPR is important in this process
- Remove jewellery from the casualty if it is in direct contact with the electrodes, or if it is in the path of one electrode to another
- Only use pads that are supplied by the manufacturer. Ensure they are in date and that the packaging is not damaged or broken
- Do not connect an AED to a casualty that is breathing normally
- Familiarise yourself with the device you have, and ensure that it has the right protocol embedded within it. If you are unsure, check with your manufacturer
- The manufacturers will have guidelines in respect of maintenance. Make sure you adhere to them
- Ensure that you use the recommended batteries as specified by the manufacturer, and that they are charged and ready to go
- Keep the pads 10cms away from any pacemaker that may be fitted
- Do not use an AED on an infant unless you have specially modified pads. If you are in doubt, you must check with the manufacturer

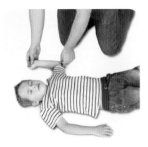

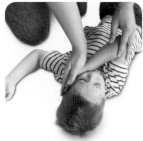

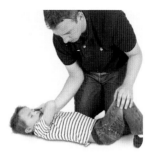

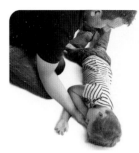

1 Place the arm nearest to you out at a right angle to their body, elbow bent with the hand palm-up. Do not force the arm, let it fall naturally, but close to this position

2 Bring the far arm across the chest, and hold the back of the hand against their cheek nearest to you

3 With your other hand, grasp the far leg just above the knee and pull it up, keeping the foot on the ground

4 Keeping their hand pressed against their cheek, pull on the far leg to roll them towards you onto their side with their head supported all the way. Adjust the upper leg so that both the hip and knee are bent at right angles

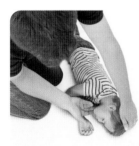

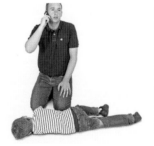

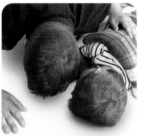

5 Tilt the head back to make sure that the airway remains open

6 Call the emergency services if you haven't yet done so

7 Check breathing regularly

If the infant is unresponsive, but breathing normally, then your priority is to ensure that their airway is not compromised in any way and that it remains open.

Rather than leaving them on their back, an effective way of achieving this is to place them in the recovery position.

Hold the infant in your arms with their head facing downwards and towards you so that you can monitor their airway, their breathing and their general condition.

If their condition deteriorates in any way, then it is vital to update the emergency services.

It is important to keep them with you at all times, particularly when contacting the emergency services.

Whilst the casualty remains in this position, it will allow vomit to drain from their mouth and maintain an open airway.

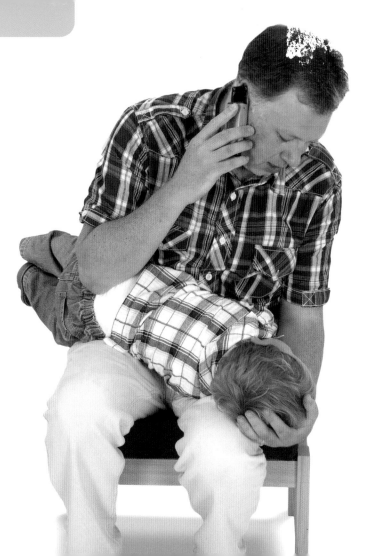